HEALTHY LIVING
WITH
HYPERTENSION

HEALTHY LIVING WITH HYPERTENSION

A GUIDE FOR AFRICAN AMERICANS

*A PRIMER FOR HIGH BLOOD PRESSURE MANAGEMENT
IN THE PRIMARY CARE SETTING*

CHERYL CAMPBELL ATKINSON PhD, RD, LDN

*These basic guidelines have been prepared primarily
for use by
non-nutrition health care professionals.*

iUniverse, Inc.
New York Lincoln Shanghai

HEALTHY LIVING WITH HYPERTENSION
A GUIDE FOR AFRICAN AMERICANS

iUniverse, Inc.

For information address:
iUniverse, Inc.
2021 Pine Lake Road, Suite 100
Lincoln, NE 68512
www.iuniverse.com

This manual is intended for informational purposes only and is not to be used in place of appropriate medical care. Health care professionals who use this manual are advised to consult with a licensed physician and or a registered dietitian before making permanent changes in the medical nutritional therapy of the clients in their care. With the availability of new research finding, high blood pressure data is ever changing. The information in this manual is the most current available.

ISBN: 0-595-33322-2

Printed in the United States of America

INTENDED USER

A PROFESSIONAL RESOURCE MANUAL

Healthy Living With Hypertension—A Guide For African Americans; A primer for high blood pressure management in the primary care setting is tailored to meet the varying educational backgrounds of most health care providers.

The medical nutrition therapy for hypertension is most appropriately designed and implemented by the skilled registered dietitian (RD). When an RD is not available, these responsibilities along with the subsequent monitoring of the patient will be the responsibility of a member of the health care team. This team member usually ends-up being a non-nutrition health professional.

This manual is designed to help the non-nutrition health professional obtain the basics necessary to provide initial counseling and/or monitoring of these patients, and in particular the African American patient with high blood pressure.

FOREWORD

As a practicing physician, with a large African American patient population, I have been impressed that many patients desire to embrace heart healthy eating, but find many of the dietary modifications and recipes in professional magazines and books unappealing. Diet and other lifestyle modifications are probably the most important things a person can do to prevent the ravages of hypertension and coronary heart disease, our nation's number one killer; and appropriate dietary counseling is the cornerstone for these changes.

'Healthy Living With Hypertension—A Guide For African Americans', provides practical nutritional advice along with tasty recipes and low sodium spices to one of the populations most affected by this disease. The author must be commended for presenting the information in such and easy-to-read and understandable way.

In the African American community, hypertension and heart disease continue to cause an unacceptable amount of death and disability. Perhaps public awareness and some of the methods highlighted in this important book will be an important step towards reducing this often-unnecessary killer.

Bruce M. Henry, MD,
St. Barnabas Hospital, New York City

Content

CHAPTER 1

INTRODUCTION

HYPERTENSION: The African American Perspective

Hypertension, commonly termed high blood pressure, is a major public health problem not just in the United States of America, but in countries world wide. The National Heart, Lung and Blood Institute's "Fact Book Fiscal Year 1996", indicates that hypertension is the second most common cause of renal problems, most noticeable end-stage renal disease, and a major cause of death in North America. Due to the asymptomatic nature of this disease it may go undetected and undiagnosed for many years in all populations at risk.

More than any other race or ethnic group, African Americans are at high risk for developing hypertension. In fact, the prevalence of high blood pressure among African Americans is among the highest in the world. The rates of hypertension in Hispanic Americans, Caucasians, and Native Americans are about equivalent (ranging from 24% to 27%. Individuals of Mexican descent, compared to Spanish descent, may have a lower risk). The rate is much lower in Asian Pacific Islanders (9.7% in men and 8.4% in women). There seems to be no definitive reason for this obvious difference in the incidence of the disease between other races and ethnic groups. The 'Well-Connected Report' March 2002, edited by Harvey Simon, MD, Editor-in-Chief, Associate Professor of Medicine, Harvard Medical School; reported that a number of theories have surfaced addressing the reasons for this difference. These theories suggest that;

- "Some studies have indicated that African Americans may have lower levels of nitric oxide and higher levels of a peptide called endothelin-1 (ET-1) than Caucasians. (Nitric oxide keeps blood vessels flexible and open and ET-1 narrows blood vessels.)

- African Americans have a higher risk for an impaired response to angiotensin (Ang II), which is a peptide important in regulating salt and

1

water balances. (African Americans are more likely to be salt-sensitive than other groups.)

- income disparities and dietary issues may explain many of the differences in blood pressure rates observed between ethnic groups. In any case, inadequately controlled hypertension is the major factor for the higher mortality rate from heart disease among African Americans".

The United States is a melting pot of many cultures from around the world. This cultural diversity impacts what and how we eat. Although African Americans now live in every state in the land, the lifestyle of parents and grandparents, who lived primarily in the southern United States, had the greatest influence on creating the social, religious and cultural traditions practiced by African Americans. These traditional practices, which have survived through today, have at their center, soul food cooking and feasting with family and friends.

'Soul Food' is a term coined by African Americans to capture the uniqueness of the cooking style utilized by themselves, families and friends, all prepared with love, care and lots of soul. These foods differ from the more traditional southern foods in the use of plain ingredients, inexpensive cuts of meat, and seasonally grown or freshly caught foods. Many of these foods are rich in vitamins and minerals, but are also rich or high in total fat, saturated fat, cholesterol and sodium (salt).

Most Americans eat too much salt in their daily diet. Some even consume up to twenty times the amount of salt needed by the body. Research indicates that diets high in salt (sodium) may cause an increase in blood pressure in many individuals. This is especially true in salt-sensitive individuals, such as African Americans. High blood cholesterol is also a risk factor for heart disease. Fortunately both high blood pressure and high blood cholesterol can be controlled in part by making some simple changes in what you eat. Cutting back on salt and sodium can help lower blood pressure. Cutting back on saturated fat and cholesterol can help lower high blood cholesterol. It is important to realize that eating fewer Kilocalories (kcal) will help lower both high blood pressure and high blood cholesterol, and control overweight at the same time.

This manual provides the non-nutrition health-care professional with ideas to assist in planning the medical nutritional therapy for hypertensive clients; cutting back on salt, as well as providing soul food recipes that are lower in sodium, fat, and cholesterol. It's all about 'heart-healthy living'.

CHAPTER 2

ASSESSMENT OF HYPERTENSION

The assessment, diagnosis and treatment of patients with hypertension is a team effort. The health care team, which is comprised of the physician, nurse, dietitian, pharmacist and other health professionals, determines the medical and the nutritional therapy to be followed, to maintain a healthy lifestyle. This process starts with a confirmed diagnosis of hypertension which is determined by measuring blood pressure.

The protocol or procedural steps:

The physical examination will include blood pressure measurements

- The measurement will be taken using a sphygmomanometer, while the patient is seated.

- The health care worker taking the blood pressure listens through a stethoscope.

- The systolic and the diastolic blood pressures are recorded.

- The diagnosis of hypertension is determined by at least two elevated blood pressure readings on two or more occasions.
(Considered high; when the readings are greater than 139/89 mm Hg)

False 'low' pressure reading can be caused by:

- Recent exercise

- Not smoking—after heavy, long-term smoking

False 'high' pressure reading can be caused by:

- An arm cuff place too tightly, or one that is too small

- Talking during the test

- Consumption of coffee (caffeine containing beverages) before testing

- Stress or tension

The nutritional assessment then continues with;

Health history
Medication history
Personal history
Diet history

Additional test also help to classify the type of hypertension manifested in the patient (secondary or essential—see pg.). These tests may include, but are not limited to:

- Blood test and urinalysis
- An electrocardiogram (ECG)
- A stress test

The findings are them evaluated and the relevance to the patient's nutritional condition discussed. The appropriate treatment is then designed and implemented by the health care team.

CHAPTER 3

QUESTIONS ABOUT DIET, WEIGHT AND HIGH BLOOD PRESSURE

Q. What is blood pressure?

A. It is the force or push of blood as it flows through the blood vessels.

Q. What is high blood pressure?

A. Blood pressure normally goes up and down in response to body demands and activities. When your numbers are consistently above 139/89mm Hg *(systolic/diastolic) you are experiencing high blood pressure or hypertension (medical term for high blood pressure). Excellent blood pressure would be less than 120/80mm Hg.

> *Systolic: the systolic pressure is the first and usually the higher number, and it is the measurement of the force that blood exerts on the artery walls as the heart contracts to pump out the blood.

> *Diastolic: the diastolic pressure is the second and usually the lower number, and it is the measurement of the force as the heart relaxes to allow the blood to flow into the heart.

> *mm Hg: Blood pressure is measured in millimeters of mercury.

Q. What are some facts about high blood pressure?

A. One out of every four Americans has high blood pressure. One out of every three African Americans has high blood pressure. High blood pressure has no clear symptoms. A person can have high blood pressure and not know it. High blood pressure cannot be cured, but it can be controlled.

Hypertension is classified in two ways;

Essential or primary hypertension:
Ninety five percent (95%) of all persons diagnosed will be in this group. Essential hypertension is of unknown etiology, but is positively influenced by modified behavioral patterns and dietary intake.

Secondary hypertension:
The remaining five percent (5%) of all persons diagnosed will be in this group. Secondary hypertension is less common, and is usually present because of some other medical condition such as renal, endocrine or neurologic disorders.

Q. **Does what we eat affect blood pressure?**

A. Yes. Eating foods that are very high in salt can increase the blood pressure in people who are sensitive to it.

Q. **What do we know about weight and high blood pressure?**

A. High blood pressure is more common in overweight people. As a person gains weight, blood pressure tends to rise; when a person loses weight, blood pressure often goes down.

    About one-third of patients with high-blood pressure are overweight. Even if the patient is moderately obese, he/she will have double the risk of hypertension than the patient with a normal weight.

Q. **Will maintaining a healthy weight prevent high blood pressure?**

A. No one knows for sure, but maintaining a healthy weight may reduce the risk of getting high blood pressure. In fact blood pressure rises as body weight increases.

    • There are two methods used to determine if one is of healthy weight; the BMI (Body Mass Index) and Waist circumference.

- 'BMI' measures the weight relative to the height, but may over or under estimate body fat.
- 'Waist circumference measurement' checks abdominal fat. A waist measurement of more than 35 inches in women and more than 40 inches in men is considered high—increases the risk of hypertension.

Q. **What is the best way to lose weight?**

A. The best way to lose weight is to eat a variety of foods each day; reduce the fat and sugar content of your diet by replacing desserts and snacks with fruits and vegetables; and include some type of exercise, like a vigorous walk, in your daily routine. A BMI less than 25 is ideal, and supports a heart healthy lifestyle.

- BMI of 25 to 29.9 -   Overweight
- BMI of 30 or greater -   Obese

Q. **How much sodium is too much?**

A. A reasonable amount of sodium in the diet of the average person is 2 grams (2000 mg) daily, which is equal to the amount of sodium found in 1 teaspoon of salt. Most Americans eat 2 to 4 times more sodium than they need by salting their foods and eating foods high in sodium.

- FYI: Table Salt

Table salt is a mixture of two substances—sodium and chloride. There is 40 percent sodium and 60 percent chloride in table salt. One teaspoon of salt = 2000 mg. sodium.

Q. **What about using salt substitutes?**

A. If you want to use salt substitutes, choose those that do not contain potassium chloride (KCl). There are several brands available. Ask your doctor before you make a decision to try salt substitutes.

Q. Are there specific diets for people with high blood pressure?

A.   No but doctors and dietitians often provide calorie and sodium controlled diets, tailored to each person's medical condition, food preferences and lifestyle. Dietitians and Nutritionists can also give tips on how to shop for appropriate foods, and how to prepare tasty meals with little or no salt.

> The DASH (Dietary Approach to Stop Hypertension) Diet is now often recommended as the principle diet therapy in managing blood pressure. The RD is the healthcare professional best trained to design and manage The diet, but when an RD is unavailable, the following recommendations

- Avoid saturated fat
- When choosing fat, select monounsaturated oils, such as olive or canola oils
- Choose whole grains over white flour or pasta products
- Choose fresh fruits and vegetables every day, especially those that are rich in fiber; (lowers blood pressure) and potassium; and Vitamin C;(boost the effects of calcium-channel blocking drugs.
- Include nuts, seeds or legumes (dried beans & peas) daily.
- Choose modest amounts of protein
  - Fish: especially oily fish is beneficial because they contain omega-3 fatty acids.
  - Soy: in combination with fiber-rich foods

Supplements which may have specific benefits should be presented to the patients.

Changing eating habits can be a fun challenge, but it takes time. Friends and family of patients can help by being supportive in an effort to help them make permanent changes towards a healthier lifestyle.

Source: adapted from the Manual of Clinical Dietetics—6th Edition, 2000
Source: adapted from NIH publications No.-2024, September 1987; and 88–1459 September 1988.

CHAPTER 4

PROTOCOL FOR HYPERTENSION DIET THERAPY

Hypertension or high blood pressure cannot be cured in most cases, but it can be effectively managed, therefore providing a better quality of life for the patient.

The medical therapy for this disease requires lifestyle changes involving diet and medication.

The medical nutrition therapy plan for the hypertensive patient is best accomplished using the specialized skills of a registered dietitian (RD). When the RD is unavailable the dietary guidance of the patient may fall on other member of the health care team. The following nutrition therapy plans should be used to initiate and or monitor the diet until the RD is able to do so.

The National High Blood Pressure Education Program (NHBPEP) recommends a diet that contains 2000–2400 mg. sodium (approximately 1 teaspoon salt), for patients with hypertension. The DASH (Dietary Approach to Stop Hypertension)—sodium study however, showed greater results with a diet that had a sodium content of 1500 mg. daily.

The DASH DIET is now often recommended as the principal diet therapy in managing blood pressure. It is recommended that patients:

- Avoid saturated fat
- When choosing fat, select monounsaturated oils, such as olive or canola oils
- Choose whole grains over white flour or pasta products
- Choose fresh fruits and vegetables every day, especially those that are rich in Fiber (lowers blood pressure) and Potassium; and Vitamin C (boost the effects of calcium-channel blocking drugs).
- Include nuts, seeds or legumes (dried beans & peas) daily.
- Choose modest amounts of protein

  o Fish: especially oily fish is beneficial because they contain omega-3 fatty acids.
  o Soy: in combination with fiber-rich foods or supplements may have specific benefits and should be presented to the patient.

Serving sizes used with the High Blood Pressure Diet—DASH

Diet based on 2000 Kcal, and 1500 mg Sodium daily.

Grain	7 – 8 servings
Vegetables	4 – 5 servings
Fruits	4 – 5 servings
Low fat or Fat-free Dairy	2 – 3 servings
Meats, poultry & Fish	2 or less servings
Nuts, seeds & Dry beans	4 – 5 servings per week
Fats & Oils	2 – 3 servings
Sweets	5 servings per week

To assist the patient with adhering to the low sodium diet lifestyle, a list of special considerations have been generated and should be used as the steps to success when teaching or counseling.

The following guide may be copied and used as a handout.

<u>Steps to Success—Low Sodium Diet Lifestyle.</u>

Read Food Labels	Check the nutrition facts label for sodium content.
Limit Consumption of High-Sodium Processed Food	Includes pre-packaged, frozen and canned foods
Remove the Salt Shaker from the Table	Refrain from purchasing salt at the grocery
Add Flavor with Herbs And Spices	These all add flavor without adding sodium
Beware of Salt Substitutes	Read the labels, and if taking blood pressure medication, consult your physician before using the substitute
Maintain a Healthy Body Weight and Exercise Regularly	Regular exercise is important in helping to lose weigh and maintain weight loss. It also keeps blood pressure down.
Alcohol in Moderation	Consume no more than one ounce per day
Eat Potassium-rich Foods	Works in concert with sodium to regulate blood pressure.

One Day Sample menu: approximately 1500 mg sodium

BREAKFAST:

½ c.	orange juice
1 c.	Oatmeal
1 c.	Skim (or fat-free) milk
2 sl.	Whole wheat toast with low-sodium margarine
1 med.	Banana
1 c.	decaffeinated coffee

LUNCH:

½ c.	fruit cup (natural juices)
3 ozs.	grilled Chicken breast
½ c.	grilled Zucchini
½ c.	Pasta salad with low-sodium dressing
1 sl.	Italian Bread
1 tsp.	Low-sodium margarine
1 c.	skim (fat-free) milk

DINNER:

4 ozs.	Halibut or Trout (broiled)
½ c.	Broccoli
2	Boiled potatoes with parsley
1	whole wheat roll
1 tsp.	Low-sodium margarine
1 c.	mixed lettuce greens with oil & vinegar dressing
½ c.	sherbet
1 c.	decaffeinated coffee

SUBSTITUTION SUGGESTIONS: Retain that 'down-home' taste

RATHER THAN:	TRY:
1 cup butter	7/8 cup vegetable oil, or 1 cup tub margarine, or 1 cup (2 sticks) margarine
1 cup heavy cream	1 cup evaporated skim milk
1 medium whole egg	2 egg whites
2 egg yolks	1 whole egg
1 cup whole milk	1 cup skim milk
1 cup sour cream	1 cup plain low-fat yogurt
1 ounce baking chocolate	3 Tbsp. Cocoa powder blended with 1Tbsp. Vegetable oil
1 cup mayonnaise	1 cup low Kcalorie salad dressing
Neck bone	skinless chicken thighs
Pork sausage	Ground skinless turkey breast
Ground beef or pork	Ground skinless turkey breast
Pork bacon	Turkey bacon, Lean ham

CHAPTER 5

DIET—DRUG INTERACTIONS

Food and Drugs (or medication) interact in various and complex ways. Foods eaten may have an effect on the medications given, causing the medication to become more powerful causing an interference with the body's ability to absorb nutrients.

It is important to understand the interaction of food with the prescribed medication because some clients may experience loss of appetite, dry mouth, weight gain, weakness, nausea, diarrhea or constipation.

GENERAL INFORMATION:

If the patient has been prescribed a hypertensive medication suggest the following;

- Medication is taken at the same time every day
- Follow the directions regarding taking the medication with or without food
- Do not eat salty foods or add salt to the food
- Consume a diet with adequate calories
- Eat fruits and vegetables, especially those high in potassium, daily. Many hypertensive medications remove potassium from the body.

When a diuretic (fluid pill) has been prescribed, suggest the following;

- Take the medication at the same time every day
- If the diuretic upsets the stomach, take it with food
- Avoid high—sodium (salt) foods
- Eat fruits and vegetables, especially those high in potassium, daily.
- Avoid using potassium-containing salt substitute
- Avoid sodium-containing antacids
- Drink a low-fat milk/milk product daily to help increase calcium and vitamin D, reducing the risk of osteoporosis

There are many medications prescribed to help lower blood pressure. With new medications becoming available constantly, a listing of the names of the drugs available in the marketplace would become incomplete almost daily. All medications fall into nine main categories however, and each category works in various ways.

Many patients will be taking two or more types of prescribed medication to bring their pressure down to a health level.

CATEGORY OF MEDICATION	WHAT DOES IT DO
**Diuretics	Called 'water pills'. They flush excess water and sodium through the kidneys, and remove them from the body in the urine.
Beta-blockers	Makes the heart beat less often and with less force by reducing the nerve impulses sent to the heart and blood vessels. The blood pressure drops, and the heart works less hard.
Angiotensin converting enzymes inhibitors	Prevents the formation of a hormone called angiotensin11, which normally causes blood vessels to narrow. The blood vessels relax, and pressure goes down.
Angiotensin antagonists	These protect blood vessels from angiotensin11. As a result the blood vessels open wider, and pressure goes down.
Calcium channel blockers	Keep calcium from entering the muscle cells of the heart and blood vessels. Blood vessels, allowing blood to pass more easily.
Alpha-blockers	Allows blood to pass more easily through the blood vessels by reducing nerve impulses.
Alpha-beta-blockers	Combines the function of the alpha-blocker and the beta-blocker: reduces nerve impulses to blood vessels and also slows the heartbeat.
Nervous system inhibitors	These relax blood vessels by controlling nerve impulses.
Vasodilators	These directly open blood vessels by relaxing the muscle in the vessel walls

Source: adapted from *Manage your Blood Pressure Drugs*

Additional Information:

**For African Americans.
- Diuretics; respond well to these drugs
- ACE inhibitors are effective and also protect the kidneys
- Calcium-channel blockers are often, they are very expensive

Patients with Diabetes:
- need to control their blood pressure to 130/85 mm Hg or lower to protect the heart and help prevent other complications common to both diseases.
- ACE inhibitors are the first
- Combinations are required to achieve blood pressure goals

Patients with Obesity:
- Losing weight is critical,
- Some newer and effective weight-loss agents, such as sibutramine (Meridia), may actually raise blood pressure.
- ACE inhibitors and angiotensin receptor blockers may be helpful

REMEMBER:
Recommend to all patients to;

- Take the medication as prescribed
- Some over-the-counter drugs can raise your blood pressure because of the high sodium content. Make a habit of carefully reading the labels of all over-the-counter drugs. Check for the sodium content. Be cautious of;
  - Arthritis medications
  - Pain medications
  - Dietary supplements (ephedra, ma haung, bitter orange)
  - Antacids; containing more than 5 milligrams

'Helpful—Tips'

To help patients remember to take their medication suggest that they:

- Put the blood pressure medication on the night stand next to the bead

- Put the medication in a weekly pillbox

- Ask a child or grandchild to remind you daily

- Put a reminder note in a visible place; refrigerator, mirror, bedroom door

- Set up a buddy system with someone with hypertension

CHAPTER 6

OTHER NUTRIENTS AND BLOOD PRESSURE

FIBER

The benefits of a high-fiber diet are dramatic in persons with high blood pressure. An emphasis on fresh vegetables, fruits, and whole grain cereals, breads, and pastas are important, since these are high fiber foods. Fiber helps to modulate the amount of salt consumed, therefore helping to prevent hypertension and the metabolic results of hypertension: kidney and heart disease.

POTASSIUM

Dietary potassium may play a role in decreasing blood pressure. Increasing potassium in the diet may protect against hypertension in people who are sensitive to high levels of sodium. The American Heart Association recommends a sodium-to-potassium ratio of one-to-one, or equal amounts of sodium and potassium. However, taking potassium supplements is generally not recommended for people with high blood pressure. Instead, a variety of potassium-rich foods should be eaten daily.

ALCOHOL

Ten percent of hypertension cases are caused by alcohol abuse. Moderate drinking however, (one or two drinks a day) has benefits for the heart and may even protect against some types of stroke; but even low or moderate drinking may increase the risk for hypertension in African Americans. Red wine specifically may have chemicals that benefit blood pressure. (Red grape juice may have the same advantages)

CAFFEINE

Caffeine causes a temporary increase in blood pressure. Regular, heavy coffee consumption (an average of 5 cups per day) will boost blood pressure, and may be harmful in people with hypertension and may even increase their risk for stroke.

HERBAL SUPPLEMENTS

Herbal supplements are often used to treat hypertension; however, they have serious side effects if taken in large doses. It is recommended that these herbs be used only under the supervision of a physician.

- **Coleus forskohlii**—Lowers blood pressure and improves heart function.
- **Hawthorne**—Has the ability to dilate coronary blood vessels, which helps lower blood pressure.
- **Mistletoe**—Not as potent as Rauwolfia but well tolerated and nontoxic in normal doses.
- **Rauwolfia**—This is considered the most powerful hypotensive botanical. Only a small dose is required to achieve results and to avoid side effects. Nasal congestion is the most common side effect.

Source: *Cardiology Channel; Hypertension*

CHAPTER 7

HERBS & HERBAL SHAKERS

Most Americans, especially African Americans and the Elderly are sensitive to salt and sodium, and usually use more of these substances than is needed in food preparation. Salt substitutes are acceptable, if approved by the doctor, but better yet, try the following seasonings with your favorite foods. These herbal seasonings also make a great flavor booster when combined and used as an herbal shaker.

Spice it up!!!

Herbs & Spices	Uses
Allspice	Lean meats, stews, Tomatoes, apple sauce, Gravies, peaches
Basil	Lean meat, Fish, Lamb, Salads, Soups, Sauces
Bay Leaves	Lean meat, Stews, Poultry, Soups, Tomatoes
Caraway Seeds	Lean meats, Stews, Salads Breads, Noodles, Soups
Chives	Salads, Sauces, Soups, Lean meat, Cabbage, noodles
Cinnamon	Salads, Vegetables, Fruits, Breads, Snacks, Piecrust
Chili Powder	Fish, Soups, Salads
Curry Powder	Lean meats, Veal, Chicken, Fish, tomatoes, Soup

Cloves	Soups, Ham, Salads,
Dill (weed & seed)	Soups, Beef, Lamb, Chicken, Fish, vegetables, Salads
Garlic	Lean meat, Fish, Soups, Salads, Vegetables, Pork
Ginger	Lean meats, Salads, Chicken, Fruits, Beverages
Lemon/Lime Juice	Fish, Salads, Vegetables
Mace	Hot breads, Apples, Veal, Lamb, Vegetables, Salads
Marjoram	Beef, Fish, Chicken, Soups, Salads, Vegetables
Nutmeg	Fruits, Lean meats, Veal, Fish, Vegetables, Potatoes
Oregano	Soups, Salads, Tomatoes, Lean ground meat, Sauces
Paprika	Lean meats, Fish, Soups, Salads, Sauces, Vegetables
Parsley	Lean meats, Fish, Soups, Sauces
Rosemary	Chicken, Veal, Pork, Lean meat Potatoes, Sauces
Sage	Lean meats, Stews, Vegetables, Biscuits, Onions
Thyme	Lean meats, Veal, Pork, Salads, Soups, Vegetables, Tomatoes

Experiment with these herbs and spices to spice up low-sodium or salt free meals.

HERBAL SHAKERS:

Mixtures and shakers can be purchased at the supermarket but here are a few which are proven 'flavor boosters". They can be used instead of salt on many types of foods.

**For a shaker use a clean glass jar with a plastic screw top; store in a dry place.

Shaker #1

1 ½ tsp.	Thyme
1 ½ tsp.	Sage
2 tsp.	Rosemary
2 tsp.	Marjoram
2 ½ tsp.	Savory

Shaker #2

1 tsp.	Celery Seed
2 ½ tsp.	Marjoram
1 ½ tsp.	Savory
1 ½ tsp.	Thyme
1 ½ tsp.	Basil

Shaker #3

2 ½ tsp.	Paprika
2 ½ tsp.	Garlic Powder
2 ½ tsp.	Dry Mustard
5 tsp.	Onion Powder
½ tsp.	Pepper
¼ tsp.	Celery Seed
½ tsp.	Parsley Flakes

Shaker #4

2 tbsp.	Crushed Savory
1 tbsp.	Dry Mustard
1 ½ tsp.	Onion Powder
1 ½ tsp.	Curry Powder
1 ¼ tsp	White Pepper
1 tsp.	Ground Cumin
½ tsp.	Garlic Powder

Source: adapted from "Recipes for the Heart"

Shaker #5

2 tbsp.	Dillweed or Crushed Basil Leaves
1 tsp.	Crushed Oregano Leaves
2 tbsp.	Onion Powder
1 tsp.	Celery Seed
¼ tsp.	Dried Grated Lemon Peel

All Purpose Herbal Shaker

Shaker #6

5 tsp.	Onion Powder
2 ½ tsp.	Garlic Powder
2 ½ tsp.	Paprika
2 ½ tsp.	Dry Mustard
1 ½ tsp.	Thyme Leaves
½ tsp.	White Pepper
¼ tsp.	Celery Seeds

CHAPTER 8

FOOD LABELS

Sodium (salt) is found naturally in food. Processed foods however have additional sodium compounds incorporated in the product as a necessary function of processing. Processed foods (canned and in some cases frozen foods), have high levels of sodium per serving. The importance of reading the food label on all foods products purchased for consumption must be stressed to all patients especially African American patients.

Always read the label of any food product purchased and select only foods that are identified as being low in sodium.

Certain compounds that provide sodium to the diet are listed below. These products should be avoided.

Monosodium Glutamate (MSG):	use in restaurants and hotel cooking. Found in many packaged, canned and frozen foods.
Sodium Benzoate:	used as a preservative in certain condiments, like relishes, sauces and salad dressings.
Sodium Propionate:	used in pasteurized cheese and in some breads
Disodium Phosphate	used in some quick-cooking cereals and Process cheeses
Sodium Hydroxide	used in food processing to softer and loosen skins of ripe olives and certain fruits and vegetables.
Sodium Alginate	used in many chocolate milks and ice Creams to make a smooth mixture.

Source: *adopted from Shaking your salt Habit*

THE LABEL LINGO

Cooking with salt and salt containing products may seem so natural that it is done with out much notice. Patients that are salt sensitive must stop, and think before cooking. Products that are low-sodium or sodium-free must be used in place of high sodium processed foods.

What do the terms 'sodium-free', 'low-sodium' or even 'salt-free' really mean when they appear on the nutritional label?

LABEL TERMS	MEANING
Sodium free	Less then 5 milligrams sodium per serving
Very low sodium	35 milligrams or less sodium per serving
Reduced or Less sodium	At least 25% less sodium*
Light in sodium	50% less sodium* restricted to foods with more than 40 Kcalories per serving or more than 3 grams fat per serving.
Low sodium	140 milligrams or less sodium per serving
Low sodium meal	140 milligrams or less sodium per 100 grams
Salt free	Less than 5 milligrams sodium per serving
Unsalted or no added salt	No salt added during processing; does not necessarily mean sodium free

* as compared with a standard serving size of the traditional food

CHAPTER 9

SODIUM CONTENT OF POPULAR FOODS

FOOD	SERVING	SODIUM (MG)
Milk Group		
Skim Milk	1 cup	122
Buttermilk	1 cup	257
Yogurt—low fat	1 cup	159
Ice Cream- vanilla	1 cup	112
Cheeses		
Swiss	1 oz.	74
Cheddar	1 oz	176
Processed American	1 oz.	406
Parmesan	1 oz.	454
Bread & Cereal Group		
White Bread	1 slice	114
Wheat Bread	1 slice	132
Cereals		
Grits, regular	¾ cup	0
Grits, instant	¾ cup	354
Oatmeal, regular	¾ cup	1
Oatmeal, instant	¾ cup	223
Shredded Wheat	1 biscuit	3
Raisin Bran	½ cup	209
Corn Flakes	1 cup	256
Rice Krispies	1 cup	340
Crackers		
Saltine	2 crackers	70
Graham	1 cracker	48

FOOD	SERVING	SODIUM (MG)
Convenience Foods		
Cake from Mix		
Yellow	1/12 cake	242
Chocolate	1/12 cake	402
Condiments		
Italian Dressing	1 tbsp.	116
French Dressing	1 tbsp	214
Mayonnaise	1 tbsp.	78
Catsup	1 tbsp	156
Soy Sauce	1 tbsp.	1,029
Garlic Salt	1 tbsp.	1,850
Meat Tenderizer	1 tsp.	1,750
Olives, green	4	323
Pickle, dill	1 large	928
Pickle, sweet	1 large	128
Salt/Spices		
Garlic Salt	1 tsp.	1,850
Onion Salt	1 tsp.	1,620
Seasoning Salt	1 tsp.	1,620
Table Salt	1 tsp.	2,325
Basil	1 tsp.	-
Bay Leaf	1 med.	-
Oregano	1 tsp.	-
Parsley	1 tsp.	5
Thyme	1 tsp.	-
Pudding		
Regular	½ cup	73
Instant	½ cup	195
Soup—Canned		
Vegetable	1 cup	823
Tomato	1 cup	872
Mushroom	1 cup	1,076
Chicken Noodle	1 cup	1,107

FOOD	SERVING	SODIUM (MG)
Snacks		
Potato Chips	10 chips	200
Pretzels (twist)	1 pretzel	101
Peanuts, roasted	1 oz.	119
Nuts, mixed	1 oz.	189
Cheese Crackers	1 piece	20
Candy Corn	1 oz.	60
Fast Food (sandwiches)		
Burger King BK Broiler	1 serving	764
Burger King Chicken Tenders	1 piece	90.2
Burger King Breakfast Croissant	1 serving	1,080
KFC—Chicken Sandwich	1 serving	1,060

Source: adapted from "The American Heart Association"

CHAPTER 10

RECIPES

The recipes in this section are to be used as handouts for the patients.

BREAKFAST DISHES

RICH BREAKFAST BISCUITS

2 cups	All Purpose Flour
2 tsps.	Baking Powder (low sodium)
2 tbsps.	Sugar
½ cup	Corn Oil
¾ cup	Skim Milk

1) Stir flour, baking powder and sugar in a medium bowl.
2) Pour oil and skim milk into flour mixture, stir with fork until four is damp.
3) Knead gently on a floured board for about 30 seconds. Pat out to ½ inch thick.
4) Using a biscuit cutter, cut dough into rounds. Place on ungreased baking sheet.
5) Bake at 450 degrees F for 12 to 15 minutes.

Makes 16 servings
*Heart and Soul

Nutrition Information: per serving
K Calories: 90
Cholesterol: 0 milligrams
Total Fat: 3 grams
Sodium: 6 milligrams

FRUITY PANCAKES

1 cup	Fruit, chopped (apples, strawberries or blueberries)
½ tbsp.	Vegetable Oil
1	Egg White
1/3 cup	Rolled Oats
2/3 cup	All Purpose Flour
½ tbsp.	Baking Powder (low sodium)

1) Combine oil, milk, egg white and fruit in a medium bowl.
2) In a separate bowl, mix together the flour, oats, sugar and baking powder.
3) Combine both the liquid and the dry ingredients together and stir lightly. Do not over stir.
4) Coat griddle with the non-stick vegetable spray.
5) Cook at 300 deg. F (medium) heat until pancakes bubble. Flip over and cook for approximately one minute. Serve hot.

Makes 4 – 6 (3" x 3") pieces

Nutrition Information: per serving:
K Calories: 134
Cholesterol: 0 milligrams
Total Fat: 2 grams
Sodium: 13 milligrams

VEGETABLE DISHES
(INCLUDING SOUPS)

GREEN BEANS AND TOMATOES IN HERBAL SAUCE

1 1-lb pk.	Frozen Green Beans
1 cup	Fresh Tomatoes, diced

<u>Sauce</u>

1 tsp.	Olive Oil
1 tsp.	Oregano
1 tbsp.	Lemon Juice
1 tsp.	Lemon Pepper

1) Steam green beans in a pot with a small amount of water. Steam until crisp-tender.
2) Drain well. Add chopped tomatoes to the green beans.
3) Combine all the ingredients for the sauce together in a small bowl.
4) Pour sauce over vegetables and toss until coated.

Makes 8 – ¼ cup servings

<u>Nutrition Information: per serving</u>
K Calories: 21
Cholesterol: 0 milligrams
Total Fat: 0.5
Sodium: 7 milligrams

BELL PEPPERS—CREOLE STYLE

4 whole	Green "bell" Peppers, cut in half
2 tsps.	Garlic, minced
¼ cup	Celery, chopped
½ cup	Onion, chopped
¼ cup	Bell Peppers, chopped
¼ cup	Water or defatted stock
¾ lb	Ground Turkey
½ cup	unseasoned Bread Crumbs

1) Put the bell peppers in a medium pot and parboil or steam in water until soft but firm. Drain well and set aside.
2) Sautee onion, celery, peppers (chopped) and garlic in ¼ cup water. Add ground turkey to vegetables and cook until the meat is brown.
3) Drain off any fat. Stir in breadcrumbs.
4) Stuff mixture into pepper halves.
5) Bake in 350 dg. F oven for 20 to 30 minutes. Add a small amount of water to bottom of pan to prevent sticking.

Makes 8 servings.

Nutrition Information: per serving
K Calories: 83
Cholesterol: 12 milligrams
Total Fat: 1 gram
Sodium: 60 milligrams

HEARTY PUMPKIN SOUP

2 tbsps.	Water
1 medium	Onion, chopped
1–16 oz. can	Pumpkin (unsweetened)
2 cups	Chicken Broth (low-sodium)
½ tsps.	Sugar
1/8 tsps.	Cloves, ground
1 cup	Skim Milk

1) In a 2-quaart saucepan with 2 tbsps. water, sauté onions until softened, about 10 minutes.
2) Add pumpkin, broth, sugar and cloves to saucepan, mix well.
3) Bring soup to the boil then reduce the heat and simmer for 15 minutes.
4) Remove from the heat and cool slightly.
5) Puree soup in small amounts in a food blender until smooth.
6) Return the coup to the saucepan and slowly pour in and stir the milk.
7) Cook for 8–10 minutes on medium high. DO NOT BOIL. Serve hot.

Makes 5, 1 cup servings.
* The ADA Family Cookbook.

Nutrition Information: per serving
K Calories: 104
Cholesterol: 1 milligram
Total Fat: 2 grams
Sodium: 32 milligrams

MEAT DISHES

ORLEANS RED BEANS (STEW)

½ lb.	Dark Red Kidney Beans
1 qt.	Water
8 ozs.*	recooked Turkey Sausage (no added salt)
8 zs.*	Precooked Beef Pieces
1 large	Onion, chopped
1 medium	Sweet Bell Pepper, chopped
4 stalks	Celery, chopped
2	Bay Leaves
2 tbsps.	Herbal Shaker #1 (see herbal shaker section)

Black Pepper to taste

*meat necessary if a meat dish is not provided.
Best if Red Beans are soaked overnight.

1) Place beans in a pot with hot water, and bring to a boil, allowing to simmer for 1 hour.
2) Add chopped seasonings (onion, bell pepper and celery) herbal seasoning, black pepper and bay leaves to the pot.
3) If meat is being used, add bite-size pieces to the beans in the pot.
4) Simmer the entire contents in the pot for an additional hour.
5) Serve over fluffy white rice.

Makes 5 – 8 servings.

Nutrition Information: per serving
K Calories:	286
Cholesterol:	40 milligrams
Total Fat:	5 grams
Sodium:	61 milligrams

HEART HEALTHY CHILI

1 lb.	Turkey, ground
½ cup	Onions, chopped
½ cup	Sweet Green Peppers, chopped
2, 8 oz cans	Tomato Sauce (low sodium)
2 cups	Red Kidney Beans, cooked
1 cup	Water
2 tsps.	Chili Powder
1 tbsps.	Herbal Shaker #2 (see herbal shaker section)

1) In a large sauce pan, place ¼ cup of water. When the water starts to boil, place the onions and green pepper and sauté.
2) Add the ground meat to the seasonings in the sauce pan, and allow to cook for approximately 10 minutes, stirring occasionally.
3) Drain off excess liquid.
4) Add remaining ingredients.
5) Cover and simmer for 1 hour, adding extra water if needed.
6) Flavor with herbal shaker #2, or the all-purpose shaker

Makes 6, 8 oz. Servings.

Nutrition Information: per serving:
K Calories: 200
Cholesterol: 5 milligrams
Total Fat: 2 grams
Sodium: 28 milligrams

OVEN BARBEQUE PORK CHOPS

4, 4 oz.	Pork Chops, lean and trimmed
½ cup	Catsup, (low-sodium)
¼ cup	Water
1 tbsp.	Brown Sugar
4 tbsps.	Lemon Juice
2 tsps.	Shaker #6

(All-purpose herbal seasoning)
Vegetable Oil Spray

1) Evenly sprinkle the pork chops with Shaker #6 and set aside for approximately 15 minutes.
2) Preheat oven to 350 deg. F. Spray the bottom of a shallow baking pan. Place the pork chops in the pan and into the oven.
3) Brown chops for 20 minutes on each side, then drain off fat.
4) Combine all remaining ingredients in a bowl, stir and then pour the mixture over the meat.
5) Cover the baking pan with foil and simmer for 30 minutes.
6) Remove the cover and continue to simmer for 10 minutes more.
7) Add more water if sauce needs to be thinned.

Makes 4, 4 oz. servings

Nutrition Information: per serving
K Calories: 221
Cholesterol: 65 milligrams
Total Fat: 5 grams
Sodium: 40 milligrams

BEVERAGES

BERRY SMOOTHEE

1, 6 oz can	Frozen Berry Punch Juice Concentrate (Minute Maid)
1 cup	Skim Milk
1 cup	Water
½ cup	Sugar
1 tsp.	Vanilla

Ice Cubes (12)

1) Place all ingredients into a blender
2) Cover and blend until smooth.
3) Serve immediately.

Makes 6, ¾ cup servings

<u>Nutrition Information: per serving</u>
K Calories: 99
Cholesterol: 0.5 milligrams
Total Fat: 0 grams
Sodium: 21 milligrams

CRANBERRY TEA DELIGHT

2 cups	Cranberry Juice Cocktail
4	Tea Bags
2 tbsps.	Sugar
2	Cinnamon Sticks, short
12	Cloves, whole

1) Place water in a sauce pan, cover and bring to a boil.
2) Put cloves, cinnamon sticks and sugar in the boiling water. Stir to dissolve sugar.
3) Remove pan from heat. Add tea bags to the solution cover.
4) Brew for 3 minutes then remove cinnamon sticks. Brew for an additional 3 minutes. Remove tea bags.
5) Add cranberry juice cocktail to the tea and return to the heat.
6) Allow the tea to reach to a boil. Remove from the heat. Serve hot.

Makes 6, 1 cup servings

Nutrition Information: per serving
K Calories:	6
Cholesterol:	0 milligrams
Total Fat:	0 grams
Sodium:	4 milligrams

STARCH DISHES

HERBAL RICE

2 cups	Water
½ cup	Carrots, shredded
½ cup	Celery, sliced
¼ cup	Onions, chopped
1 tsp.	Garlic, Minced
2 tsps.	Shaker #4
2/3 cup	Rice, long grained

1) In medium sauce pan, combine water, carrots celery, onions, garlic and herbal seasoning. Bring to a gentle boil.
2) Reduce heat and allow vegetable to cook for 2 minutes.
3) Add uncooked rice to the sauce pan.
4) Cover and simmer for 20 minutes or until rice is tender.
5) Remove from heat, let stand for approximately 5 minutes then fluff with a fork.
6) Serve hot.

Makes 2, 6 oz servings

Nutrition Information: per serving
K Calories: 145
Cholesterol: 0 milligrams
Total Fat: 2 grams
Sodium: 23 milligrams

ORANGE SWEET POTATOES

1 lb.	Fresh, Sweet Potatoes
1 cup	Orange Juice
¼ cup	Granulated Sugar
¼ tsp.	Nutmeg
1/8 tsp.	Ginger

1) Boil sweet potatoes for 20 minutes, or until cooked but not mushy.
2) Remove from pot and slice length-wise. Place in casserole dish.
3) Mix orange juice, sugar, ginger and nutmeg together.
4) Pour over sliced sweet potatoes and bake in a moderately hot oven (300 degrees) for 30 minutes. Serve hot.

Makes 4 servings.

<u>Nutritional Information: per serving</u>
K Calories: 110
Cholesterol: 0 milligrams
Total Fat: 0 grams
Sodium: 8 milligrams

ORLEANS POTATOES

4 medium   Potatoes, peeled and cut in 4 pieces

2 tbsp.   Lemon Pepper

1 tbsp.   Parmesan Cheese

2 tsps.   Parsley, dried

Vegetable Spray

1) Boil potatoes in a medium pot.
2) Bring to the boil, reduce heat and cook for approx. 15 minutes until tender but not over cooked.
3) Remove from stove top and drain.
4) Spray shallow baking pan with vegetable spray and place potatoes evenly in pan.
5) Spray potatoes lightly with vegetable spray and sprinkle with lemon pepper and parmesan cheese.
6) Place prepared potatoes in a 375 deg. F oven for 15 minutes or until brown.

Makes 4 servings

Nutritional Information: per serving
K calories: 101
Cholesterol: 1 milligram
Total Fat: 1 gram
Sodium: 33 milligram

DESSERT DISHES

PEACH APPLE COBBLER

2 cups	Fresh or Frozen Peaches, chunks (peeled)
¾ cups	All Purpose Flour
¼ cup	Applesauce (unsweetened)
1 ½ tsps	Baking Powder (low sodium)
2/3 cup	Skim Milk
½ cup	Sugar

Vegetable Oil Spray

1) Using the vegetable oil spray, grease a 1 ½ quart casserole dish.
2) Combine flour, sugar and baking powder in small mixing bowl.
3) Slowly stir in milk then add applesauce to mixture.
4) Pour batter into casserole.
5) Sprinkle peaches evenly on top of batter.
6) Bake at 350 deg. F for about 50 minutes. Serve hot.

Makes 4, 8 oz. cup servings.

Nutrition Information: per serving
K Calories: 195
Cholesterol: 0 milligrams
Total Fat: 0 grams
Sodium: 12 milligrams

ORANGE PEANUT TEA CAKE

2 cups	All Purpose Flour
3 tsps.	Baking Powder (unsalted)
2 tbsps.	Smooth Peanut Butter (no salt added)
2	Egg Whites
1/3 cup	Skimmed Evaporated Milk
1/3 cup	Water
½ cup	Orange Marmalade
½ cup	Brown Sugar

1) In a large bowl, sift flour and baking powder (unsalted) and then combine the sugar.
2) Cut in the peanut butter to this flour mixture.
3) In a small bowl, place the milk and the egg. Beat egg mixture with a fork until thoroughly blended and then add to the flour mixture.
4) Beat for 30 seconds with spoon until well blended.
5) Pat into greased 8" x 11" x 1 ½" baking pan.
6) Bake in preheated hot oven at 400 degrees for 25–30 minutes.
7) Serve warm or cold.

Makes 12 (3" x 3") pieces

Nutrition Information: per serving
K Calories: 160
Cholesterol: 0 milligrams
Total Fat: 2 grams
Sodium: 20 milligrams

References

Anderson, J. *Potassium and Health.* Colorado State University Cooperative Extension—Nutrition Resources. August 2004

Addressing the Health Care Issue of African-Americans. *Hypertension.* www.blackhealthcare.com retrieved July 2004

Alternative-Medicine-and-Health. *Hypertension.* www.alternative-medicine-and-health.com Retrieved, August 2004.

Cardiology Channel. *Hypertension.* Health Communities. www.cardiologychannel.com Retrieved, July 2004.

Fighting Heart Disease and Stroke. *Shaking your salt habit.* American Heart Association. 2001

Fighting Heart Disease and Stroke. *High Blood Pressure in African Americans.* American Heart Association 6/2003

High Blood Pressure. www.reutershealth.com retrieved August 2004

Jackson Gastroenterology. High Blood Pressure Diet, www.gicare.com/pated.htm. Retrieved, September 2004.

Kennedy, Ron MD. *Fiber in Nutrition.* The Doctor's Medical Library. www.medical-Library.net Retrieved, September 2004

Larson Duyff, R. *Complete food and Nutrition Guide.* The American Dietetic Association. 1996

Manual of Clinical Dietetics. *Hypertension.* American Dietetic Association. 6th Edition, 2000

Munson Army Health Center. *Food and Drug Interactions* ; www.munson.amedd.army.mil. retrieved June 2004.

National Heart, Lung and Blood Institute. *Fact Book Fiscal Year 1996.* Bethesda, Maryland. U.S. Department of Health and Human Services, National Institutes of Health: 1997.

National Heart, Lung and Blood Institute. *Your Guide to Lowering Blood Pressure—Manage Your Blood Pressure Drugs.* National Heart, Lung and Blood Institute Health Information Center. www.nhlbi.nuh.gov retrieved August 2004

Roe, D. A., *Handbook on Drug and Nutrient Interactions—A problem Oriented reference Guide.* 4th Edition. The American Dietetic Association. 1989

Tsang, G., *High Blood Pressure Diet—the Dash Diet.* Healthcastle Nutrition Services www.healthcastle.com Retrieved, September 2004.

0-595-33322-2